THE
PLANT-BASED DIET

Delicious Recipes to Lose Weight, Reduce Inflammation, Reverse Disease, and Feel Great

KAREN COLE

Contents

Introduction

Congratulations on downloading *Plant-Based Diet: Delicious Recipes to Lose Weight, Reduce Inflammation, Reverse Disease, and Feel Great*—and thank you for doing so!

Many times, we hear that changing your nutrition is a scientific way to live longer, reduce your risk of disease and sickness, and even help the environment. Embarking on a new way of eating does sound like a great idea, but starting this journey is a different story. This book is a perfect start to learning how a Plant-Based Diet can be just the beginning of feeling great!

This diet plan has the following as benefits:

- Can lower your cholesterol, blood pressure, and blood sugar levels

- Can reverse or help prevent heart disease
- Can aid in a longer life
- Can help establish a healthier weight
- Can reduce the use of medications
- Can help lower costs of food
- Can make our planet better
- Can lower the risk of cancer
- Can improve symptoms of rheumatoid arthritis (RA)

Don't leave a healthier YOU to chance! Learn the balanced and simple way to begin the journey of a Plant-Based Diet!

The following chapters will discuss:

- What You'll Be Eating
- Tips for This Diet
- Food-Based Mistakes
- Basic Shopping List
- 30-Day Meal Plan
- Breakfast, Lunch, and Dinner Recipes
- Desserts and Snacks

There are plenty of books on this subject on the market—thanks again for choosing this one! Every effort was made to ensure that it is full of as much useful information as possible. Please enjoy!

What You'll Be Eating

J ust the notion of consuming more plants in place of animals is an extraordinary way to boost your longevity and endurance in your personal life. You will learn to elevate your taste buds to crave healthier foods, increase your chances at preventing disease, and balance your mood and hormones with each bite. Other reasons that you are making this switch could be for your budget, the environment, and the animals, which a plant-based diet aids. Whatever the case, you must know that you have made the right choice! Soon, you are likely to experience more well-being benefits than you could have ever imagined. The incredible health benefits are blood sugar advantages, digestion improvements, cancer prevention, and an even more energetic and happier mood. You will soon learn that every single on is thanks to all the nutrient-packed properties this diet has.

Beginning a new journey starts with equipping yourself with all of the proper information to ensure success. For this kind of change in your lifestyle, you will want to know what changes that you are making. Hence, let's first understand what the core of a Plant-Based Diet is.

Plant-based foods are becoming principal in many lifestyles today, which is why more folks are looking for methods that they can embrace facets of the plant-based lifestyle in their own everyday lives. Initially, the plant-based transition is about eating primarily fruits, vegetables, whole grains, and legumes. In your research, you will find that the basis of The Plant-Based Diet has the main focus to put emphasis on eating whole, non-processed (or as minimally processed as possible) foods—most of which are from plants and do not contain any animal ingredients. With regards to animal food products, they typically are eaten only in small amounts—if any at all.

Even before embarking on using this book, you may have already started taking certain measures such as reducing your consumption of processed foods and meat. Yes, at first, this may not seem to be as trouble-free as you would like. Someone who has had the habit of eating a good amount of processed food has consumed high amounts of fructose corn syrup, artificial sugar, sodium, and other chemicals. Don't be surprised if your body starts to crave these at the beginning of your transition.

When considering what is deemed as non-processed, remember that these are natural foods that are whole, unrefined, or with minimally refined ingredients.

As you go through your search, remember that it is all about feeling better and getting control over how food affects your body. Hence, focusing on the different tasty groups that you will be enjoying is where you should start!

Thus, when it comes to your produce, people may say that "fresh is best." It does require some research for your area because sometimes, it may not be the best option available for a number of reasons.

There are numerous things influencing the nutrients that your produce contains. The harvest date and time, the proximity of source, and the duration of the display are just some of the important fluctuating circumstances. Some others are the duration of their contact with light as well as the temperature at which they are stored. These factors have the capability to impact the nutrition extractible from these produce drastically. Now, in the huge stores wherein people typically buy their products, the general public does not have knowledge of the aforementioned factors. Moreover, considering the technology today, personally evaluating the quality of the said produce is not so simple anymore, no matter how hard you try. Hence, if it is in your power to do so, opt to purchase from small but credible sources whose methods of product acquisition are known to you. Only by then that you can try getting the best you can for your dollar.

However, let's not forget that a cost-effective way of buying produce exists through your local freezer section. It is also beneficial at times that you don't have the time to prepare food. One fact that might interest you is that the nutrients of frozen produce are relatively high. This is largely due to the fact that they are on prime condition during the time that they are taken. You can take advantage of frozen produce for out-of-season items, However, always keep in mind that like anything else, its nutritional quality still depreciates as time passes by. Hence, immediate consumption is still advised.

When you go to buy breakfast cereal, almond milk, bread (whole grain), hot sauce, and pasta, make it your habit to see its list of contents in advance—the less the contents, the better. As an example, pasta completely composed of whole grain wheat and preservative-free bread can be an option, as long as they don't have any animal products (meat by-products, dairy, or egg). If it's grain-based, check its authenticity (in terms of its actual composition). A good rule of thumb is that if the term "whole" isn't explicitly indicated, then it is most likely refined, and it's better to pass that option up.

In our ventures down the grocery aisle, picking through different products, we want also to pay attention to added salt. Usually, there's a lot of them that can be found especially from packaged items. Generally speaking, for the Plant-Based Diet to be successful, a daily sodium consumption of 1500 mg must be the maximum. To do this successfully, you shouldn't completely rely on the percentages indicated, as 2300 mg is the typically suggested intake of the said element that they use.

And finally, when reading labels, we want to make sure that you are not consuming refined sugar. There are multiple names for added sugar, so understanding what they are is important. While there may be very small amounts of added sweeteners to many of the things we may use off the shelf, the focus is to eliminate as much as possible. The more you read, the more you will learn about certain brands and their content. However, in the beginning, don't worry too much, and do the best that you can. Something to also keep in mind in your choice is the existence of various sugar classifications, which may be really far down the ingredient list.

As you have seen, there are a lot of different aspects of this diet to consider as you start the process. The key is to keep it as simple as possible for you and your lifestyle because the point is: you want to be successful and not burdened down.

Hence, when you move through this book, remember that it is all about you being in control.

Here are the FOUR main groups that you will be building your meals from:

WHOLE GRAINS – These are food products made from whole or complete grains that contain the three key parts of a seed: the bran, germ, and endosperm. Some of these are bread, cereals, pasta, brown rice, quinoa, millet, oats, barley, corn, and bulgur. The bonus of whole grain foods is that they are very filling—without the fat!

The good news about this group is that research has shown that in countries where these grains are a staple, some diseases such as diabetes, heart disease, and cancer are much less common. They are filled with important nutrients including protein, fiber, B vitamins, antioxidants, iron, zinc, copper, and magnesium, or trace minerals.

LEGUMES – These are plants that bear fruit that grow in pods which can be broken down into different subsections including beans, lentils, peas, and peanuts. Some very familiar legumes are chickpeas (also known as garbanzo beans), kidney beans, black beans, soybeans, pinto beans, and navy beans. These hearty, high protein foods are rich in calcium, iron, cholesterol-lowering soluble fiber, and even traces of omega 3 fatty acids.

FRUITS AND VEGETABLES – The obvious base of this diet that is loaded with vitamins and minerals, and is very low in fat. Like all plant foods and tubers (root vegetables), they have no cholesterol at all. For the most part, fruits and vegetables are lower in calories than many other foods, so choosing to eat more, can help to lower your overall daily calorie count.

One great thing to do is to become aware of different kinds of vegetables and fruits that you might not have been familiar with. When you do this, you really help to expand your produce horizons. This book will help you learn how to prepare them properly too. The goal being, you may have thought you didn't like a particular veggie, but making it a new way could completely change how you feel!

A great benefit of eating whole fruits and vegetables adds fiber to your diet, which fills you up and helps you maintain your weight. An added bonus is, with a variety of colors, flavors, and textures; it brings life to meals and snacks. For example, you can start eating fruit for a snack instead of cookies and/or chips. By steadily adding plant-based foods into your diet, you'll be getting your mind and body used to enjoying them!

NUTS AND SEEDS – These foods may be small but are nutrient and energy-packed—loaded with vitamins, minerals, fiber, protein, and essential fatty acids such as Omega 3 fatty acids. This nutrient is a great anti-inflammatory and great for the health of our brain, skin, hair and hormone production. Adding them to meals, snacks, and desserts makes this versatile food a great addition to a healthier eating routine.

In our recipe chapters, you will learn how easy it is to create tasty and easy meals full of these categories and more. You can have full control in replacing your tastes and habits to change your health for the better. Don't feel you have to put a time table on disentangling yourself from the behaviors and patterns you have had your whole eating life. Expect to find foods you enjoy and new methods in shopping and cooking. You will love it when this becomes your new normal!

Plant-Based Whole Food Quick Reference

- Legumes
- navy beans, peas, lentils, etc.
- Leaves
- lettuce, spinach, arugula, etc.
- Bulbs
- onion, garlic, shallots, etc.
- Roots
- beet, potato, carrot, etc.
- Flowers
- cauliflower, broccoli, etc.
- Whole Grains
- wheat, brown rice, rye, etc.
- Fruits
- tomato, orange, kiwi, etc.
- Mushrooms
- Portobello, button, shiitake, etc.
- Stems
- celery, rhubarb, asparagus, etc.
- Nuts
- almonds, walnuts, sunflower seeds, etc.

Animal-Based Food Products Quick Reference

- Dairy
- cheese, milk, yogurt, butter, etc.
- Eggs
- chicken eggs, duck eggs, etc.
- Fish & Seafood
- tuna, swordfish, shrimp, scallops, clams, etc.
- Meat
- beef, pork, lard, etc.
- Poultry
- chicken, turkey, quail, duck, etc.

2

Tips for This Diet

As with any new venture, we must always make our research. Yet, in this technological day and age, one simple search about transitioning to a Plant-Based Diet can turn into an endless vortex. Before we know it, we have in front of us way too much information—nowhere to begin and the urge to say, "Never mind."

Thus, let's not go down that road—make it simple. This is definitely a possible journey to embark on! Our job here is to help get rid of all those negative thoughts—once and for all.

As with any new thing that we do, we know first that we have to get used to the idea of something different going on in our lives. Maybe you have tried this before and didn't come off as successful as you would have liked. Usually, it is because we start off with the wrong expectations. Here, you will find comfortable ways to begin this transition. For example, you may be able to start with one or two meatless days per week and then increasing that as you got more comfortable with plant-based eating. Then, try to start replacing the dairy in your diet. Do not worry—it is way easier than you might think! Another way to take one step at a time is to start substituting the dairy in your coffee with non-dairy milk. From there, you can try to lessen cheese (or completely eliminate it if you are feeling super brave). A couple of other options to try can be to eliminate eggs and go for other great "morning protein" foods. Once you are able to tackle some of these small areas and replace more and more of your food, they will be in sync!

Humans are generally creatures of habit. We may tend to find simplicity in living our lives with uniformity. Whether it is as a parent or grandparent, an employee, or a student everyone occasionally finds themselves functioning in some kind of routine. This could eventually become what we are comfortable with- Our Comfort Zone. If ever it is suggested that we do something outside of this zone, we immediately become concerned about the dreaded "unknown," which then demonstrates a basic human flaw- a fear of discomfort.

Think back for a second in your life. Can you find that any of your most enjoyable memories to have come about when you did something outside of your comfort zone? The greatest thing about comfort zones is that with each new experience that we try, we grow the limits that we have placed in our lives. So we have to remember that each and every time we step outside of these comfort zones, they will follow us. And now applying that tot his journey you are embarking on with your health, it just takes the effort to make these new habits stick permanently.

All we have to do is look at the track record of so many in history those who made that great leap and stepped outside of their comfort zone and tried something new. People like Thomas Edison or even the amazing band The Beatles were the ones who made a big impact on our world. They took advantage of the ability to revolutionize the lives of others. Yet, in a simplest of thoughts, it really isn't necessary to be in the world's spotlight to go outside of your comfort zone. Can you imagine the impact you will have on the lives around you when you are feeling healthier? Starting a plant-based diet dependent on whole plant foods has been shown to reduce the risk of lifestyle-related diseases—diabetes, heart disease, hypertension, and even certain types of cancer. What about for the future you? There's been new research that indicates that plant-based diets could be helpful in preventing Alzheimer's, Multiple Sclerosis, and lots of other degenerative diseases. And if that's not enough of a reason, minimally processed plant-foods greatly benefit our planet and its environment.

Here are 7 basic tips for making this diet a success.

Educate

When making this decision to switch, you might have a reason in mind. One of which could be for health reasons. If so, make sure you are noting just how you will be able to get the most nutrients out of what you are eating. Spend some time getting familiar with some of the different foods you will be adding to your diet. Especially so if there are some that you may not be familiar with. Have you not been a huge veggie and fruit person? Have you ever had some things only one way, which you didn't actually enjoy? This type of exploration will help you to know what you are in for. Some of us have our own preferences on what we eat on a regular basis. This journey is going to make you step out of your comfort zone. Yet, it need not be to put a frown on your face. Learn what different types of flavors can be created with certain veggies. For example, you may not have known that some plant-based foods can be cooked in ways that remind us of meat. Like portabella mushrooms, beans, jackfruit, and even tofu! DO you have a hard time letting go of sugary flavors? You would be surprised to find out how many ripe fruits can add just the right amount of sweet to our sweet tooth treats! Again, it's this type of initial education that will help gear you to be successful and not miss the bad stuff.

Also remember, everyone is different, and each plan is

different for everyone. You may have to start small and play around with different things to make it work for your lifestyle and NOT compare it to someone else or to what you may have done before.

Motivation

Changing your eating reasons is a good start. You may know that sometimes, when we experience negative emotions, we have the tendency to eat—usually, it's our most favorite treat, which can be unhealthy. This is because the brain typically responds to foods rich in calories that cause us to release "happiness hormones" (serotonin and dopamine.) As a consequence, these calorie-packed foods activate a cycle of potential addiction and possibly weight gain. The way out is to disrupt this cycle and start properly feeling great!

How many times have we started and stopped something new solely for the reason that we just weren't motivated? Adjustments in our ways of eating can definitely fall in this category. Especially if we chose to go "cold turkey." The beauty of this type of change is you are in full control of how much or how little you can adjust. If you chose the "all in, go big or go home" approach, you would immediately jumpstart your bodies accepting the new and great nutrients that it's now getting. It can even create instant accountability once all your friends and family get wind of this wonderful change. They may even join you. The key is, find what drives your motivation and lean on that, especially in the beginning stages. Especially because realistically you would like to be able to continue this diet for the rest of your life. So just do the best you can. Do not let what you eat to be a source of stress or restriction. Whichever way that you decide to take on this transition, you must do the best you can with what you have.

Start Slow

For those not so externally motivated, you may need smaller steps. Which aren't so bad, because there are some drawbacks that can be avoided by doing it gradually. Again, everyone is different, and when drastically changing your diet, you can begin to detox. This may not sound too bad in theory, especially if you know you need to rid your body of some toxins. Sometimes, though, abruptly taking major staples out of your diet can make it more likely that you'll get off track. Make sure that you have enough resources to get you started so you don't feel overwhelmed. For example, for your first plant-based meal, you may want to plan something easy so that you don't put added pressure on yourself to make a meal too complicated.

Like most lovers of what's good getting rid of the bad food is easier said than done. Nonetheless, keeping the temptations nearby only makes it more likely to give into them. But don't do it! It's impossible to resist once our brain seeks that rush we get, the rush of indulgence that bad food gives us. No matter how problematic it might appear, you have to encircle yourself only with healthy plant-based food as much as possible. Reorganize your kitchen, throw away the junk food and try to replace with healthy choices!

In the world we live in we have become accustomed to eating on the run. Typically, we eat fast food, taking one big bite after the other like we only have a short amount of time to eat while standing. Believe it or not, this bad eating behavior can teach the brain that fast is better. In term does not do well for our bodies. So we need to sit down and take our time, electing healthy plant-based meals.

For a lot of people, it is difficult to keep focused on the right track, if there is no motivation. Sure, the ultimate goal is to eat healthier, lose weight, and feel great but we cannot achieve all of these things in the blink of an eye. A good source of motivation is creating a goal calendar, with a number of targets to be achieved. Before you know, you will achieve what you want on this journey.

Talk About It

Whenever we make a change, we find friends and family will have questions. Depending on your personal life this may present a challenge, or it may be a motivation. Most times if we just put ourselves in their shoes we can understand. Maybe you have decided to bring a plant-based side dish for your contribution to family dinner. It takes courage to do that! A great start to creating this lifestyle is getting all the support you can get. So talk about it! Take the opportunity to help someone else try the new recipe that you love making. Alternatively, you may want to bring up the topic whenever you talk with your loved ones so that they aren't surprised when you add a plant-based meal to the menu. You may be surprised at how many people have been just like you. Just by you being courageous enough to embark on this journey, even if alone, you never know how many are watching and wanting to take the same courageous step in wanting to take control of their health!

Also, you never know how many are already doing it. Just like there are support groups for every aspect of life, you can have one too. Don't think that you have to gout and find the nearest group—when all you have to do is talk about this change. People of like mind always find each other. What's amazing about this is that the more you can find that under-stand, the easier it will be to stick it out. Not only will you find people who have made a success of the transition, but you will even learn more about it. And they will love to share their secrets with you! All in all, when you build up your support system, you get what you need to keep going. There will be days when it will be challenging, so utilize these ones in your life to get you back in a positive mindset.

Healthy Choices

One great way to get the ball rolling is to start making healthier choices. Especially after you begin to educate your-self on what types of foods you will be enjoying. Start looking to eat them right away! Headed out to eat with the family? Chose a plant-based side on the menu! Grabbing your usual latte at your favorite coffee shop? Try changing your order just a little bit. These little steps will make you see how easy it will become at incorporating healthy, plant-based foods in your routine every single day.

Colorful food is a healthy way to appeal to the brain. It reinforces the idea that colorful, healthy meals are the absolute best. So don't hesitate to use plenty of fresh veggies and fruits in your meals as you transition. You will be surprised to find that you can inspire yourself! You may even be inspired by the handiworks of famous cooks and look for creative ways to indulge in this new eating journey. When you use fun garnishes, fresh herbs, and aromatic spices, you will add so much life to your meals and your taste buds.

What matters most is that we stay focused, while embracing the array of variety we can have in our meals. It has been said that the brain likes to be entertained so that it looks forward to each meal. The brain is excited about a meal that is healthy, believe it or not. It releases happiness hormones, and soon you will forget all about that none plant-based food! And the thing is we do have a lot of great choices available. We have to opt for colorful veggies and fruits, incorporate different textures, and play with flavors as we wish to have great meals.

There's no denying it—sometimes, vegetables just don't cut it. But when you make an effort to turn it into a delectable, flavorful dish, you suddenly gain a new outlook on them. Comfort food can be healthy! All that's needed is some encouragement. From there you will be sure to come up with amazing and appealing dishes. How about making "fries" in the oven, enjoying a delicious ice cream made from bananas and take delight in dark chocolate. It all matters how you let yourself look at things!

Lessening your portion size is also one of the ways to jump-start this change. Initially, it may be a challenge to achieve, as we are constantly bombarded by super-large portions, especially in restaurants. Hence, when preparing your meals, try out a smaller portion. Trick your brain into opting for a portion that is smaller in size in relation to foods that may not be as healthy for us. This is guaranteed to have the envisioned effect.

Set Up Your Kitchen Right

One great way to help with the transition is to have your kitchen set up just right. Creating an atmosphere that makes cooking pleasurable; less frustrating and like a chore. You want it to be a space where you can walk in to feel inspired, creative, and determined to stick to this Plant-Based journey!

A great way to begin is with organizing your space. A very simple start can be to place a fruit bowl on the counter. Put bright colored fruit in it to help motivate your plant-based eating. And of course, this makes for easy access to some of your favorite fruits on the go. Do you love being able to find all of your spices in one place? You may want to consider creating one easy –to- reach a place near the stove for these, and your oils. If you are adventurous, maybe get a small indoor fresh herb garden to have at your fingertips. The smell alone could trigger the cooking motivation you will need!

Next, it may be time to stock up! Whether you are doing a slow transition or a full on one, having the right food in the house is key. In your efforts to get organized, do an inventory of what you already have, and also how much you can realistically store.

Another aspect of inventory can be what kitchen tools and appliances you have. This diet is supposed to be encouraging, yet if we aren't equipped with what we need to make that exciting new dish, our motivation can swiftly fade. Small things like a great pot set, skillets, cutting boards, baking sheets, and baking dishes can go a long way. Something not to overlook is a nice set of knives, and veggie choppers/peelers. These can make prep time a breeze!

Other options really depend on your budget, space, and affinity for appliances. A food processor, slow cooker, rice maker, high-speed blender, immersion blender, waffle iron, or spiralizer; are all very good to have handy at some point throughout this journey! Yet, don't fret—these types of preparations come in time, especially the more you enjoy incorporating your new eating habits to your daily routine.

Have Fun

At the end of the day, nothing is going to happen overnight. So actually enjoying the journey is essential! There may be days when you will crave something 'non-plant-based,' and that's okay. You may discover that you love bacon way more than you realized. You may even have accidentally ordered steamed milk in your latte. All hope is NOT lost! Remember, this is a journey that requires you just to put one foot in front of the other. Your way of doing that may be different than someone else. So be kind to you, recognize big or small progress and FORGIVE yourself. Most importantly, always keep going!

3

Food-Based Mistakes

As you begin to make changes, stock up on all the necessities, and move successfully through your journey—it is important to know how to avoid making some common mistakes. These can be in regards to what you eat and what you do throughout the transition.

One of the biggest initial mistakes is feeling like you won't get enough protein and yet forgetting that vegetables have protein too. All it takes is researching how many nutrients are in the plant-based foods that you consume. For example, did you know that beans, legumes, and lentils have about 13 grams of protein per cup? Likewise, did you know that 100 calories of broccoli have 11 grams of protein, while 100 calories of steak only have 8 grams of protein? Also, quinoa, soybeans, edamame, and chickpeas can average over 15 grams of protein per cup. Thus, as long as you are eating enough of the right plant-based foods throughout the day, protein won't be an issue. There are also many creative ways to fill your plate with whole food meatless options such mushrooms, jackfruit, tofu, or tempeh. It is better to create a healthier alternative to get the nutrients you need than going without on without them and later on suffering the consequences.

In line with that thought, it should be noted that if we are too restrictive with ourselves, this could be more burden-some than helpful. It's so easy to get carried away when we start cutting out certain foods or cutting back on some. Again it is important to research and apply certain changes to your own personal circumstance. For example, one Plant-Based Dieter may remove all gluten, soy and wheat products assuming they are bad for them without receiving medical advice. Yet, others may have been advised to refrain from these foods due to allergies and sensitivities. In studies by the Academy of Nutrition and Dietetics, if planned appropri-ately, a plant-based diet is nutritionally adequate and helps prevent disease. Hence, just taking control of your health by doing this is going to help fix any health concerns right from the start. So instead of creating a not so positive transition by placing too much restriction on yourself, relish in the joy of every change you make.

Another common mistake is opting for the "alternative" pre-made food options. Although they can be convenient and accessible, they may not be the healthiest choice. Again it requires research. Checking labels and contents are important. Some of the alternative food products contain high amounts of sugar, sodium, fats, and calories. This can be counter-productive to your transition. So the key with all label reading is to be able to read the actual ingredients, and that there aren't too many of them.

A way that may cause someone to fall into using these alternatives is from not planning ahead. Think of those moments when you suddenly find yourself hungry. Not planning ahead could mean not finding any accessibly healthy options or making a bad food choice. A way around to it may be choosing a specific day to prepare your meals for the week—making sure also to prepare on-the-go snacks and meals. This way, you are never stuck at the proverbial fork in the road, choosing between eating and going hungry. When choosing a day to prep and grocery shop ahead of time, you can feel stable setting up your week of eating the right way.

Lastly, one mistake that everyone can say they make—whether embarking on a new diet or not—is forgetting to drink enough water! In this case, it is very important to do so because a lot of the plant-based foods contain fiber. Since you will be consuming more than you may have in the past, staying hydrated keeps the fiber moving through the digestive tract. It will also help to avoid becoming bloated or constipated. Water is good for you and your digestive system, so do not be afraid to drink up!

4

Basic Shopping List

Below, you will find an example idea of what you should be considering as a shopping list. This can easily be used as a guide, wherein as you continue to transition, you will find your favorites!

Produce

Kale

Spinach

Collard Greens

Swish Chard

Potatoes

Broccoli

Beets

Brussels Sprouts

Carrots

Zucchini

Cucumbers

Asparagus

Red, Yellow, Orange, and Green Peppers

Avocado

Sweet Potato

Onions

Chili Peppers (Sweet and Hot)

Sprouts

Green Onions

Yams

Tomato (any variety)

Mushrooms

Bananas

Apples

Watermelon

Lemons

Limes

Peaches

Kiwi

Oranges

Tangerines

Strawberries

Raspberries

Cranberries

Blackberries

Blueberries

Grapefruit

Pineapple

Garlic

Ginger

Cilantro

Parsley (Flat and Italian)

Mint

Dill

Basil

Thyme

Large-Quantity Items

Grains - Brown Rice, Quinoa, Farro, Oats, Bulgur, Barley, etc.

Dry Beans - Black, Navy, Garbanzo, Kidney, etc.

Seeds - Chia, Flax, Pumpkin, Sunflower, etc.

Nuts - Cashews, Almonds, Walnuts, Pecans, Peanuts, etc.

Flour - Coconut, Almond, Whole Wheat

Lentils

Refrigerator and Freezer Items:

Non-Dairy Milk (unsweetened)

Non-Dairy Butter Substitute

Tempeh

Tofu

Miso

Organic & Vegan Frozen Prepared Meals

Frozen Veggies

Frozen Fruit

Canned Items

Tomatoes

Tomato Paste

Tomato Sauce

Prepared Vegan Soups

Beans - Black, Kidney, and Pinto

Pantry Items

Olives

Coconut Oil

Olive Oil

Grapeseed Oil

Avocado Oil

Tahini

Almond Butter

Peanut Butter

Cashew Butter

Whole Grain Crackers

Soba Noodles

Corn Tortillas

Whole Wheat Tortillas

Corn Tortilla Chips

Vinegar - Apple Cider, Balsamic, White Wine, and Red Wine

Plant-Based Protein Powder

Unsweetened Cocoa Powder

Spices

Hot Sauce

Coconut Flakes (unsweetened)

Whole Grain/Dijon Mustard

Nutritional Yeast

Dried Fruit

Seaweed

Pure Maple Syrup

Extracts - Vanilla, Mint, Orange, etc.

Coffee/Tea

Seltzer/Sparkling Water

5

30-Day Meal Plan

One of the hardest things to organize when transitioning into a new way of eating is an easy-to-follow meal plan. Believe it or not, Meal planning is going to improve your plant-based life by saving you time (and money) while lowering your stress! Just imagine not having that dreaded moment of standing in front of the fridge, trying to figure out what plant-based meal you are going to make for dinner. Some of the great benefits of this type of preparation are actually seeing things laid out for you so that you know where to start. Here, you will find a nice guide to use based on the recipes listed at the end of this book. As has been mentioned, everything can be customized and structured for each person.

In chapter three, we talked about common mistakes that are made in regards to our food—one being the failure to plan ahead. By using this guide, you can see that you can incorporate Meal Planning into the schedule. Although the concept might sound scary, planning meals in advance can be easy and fun! Do n0t be afraid to adjust your recipe quantities to fit your eating needs. Try not to feel over-whelmed—believing that you need to have incredible amounts of free time, lots of money, or some kind of fancy kitchen tools and appliances to make it happen. When you plan ahead, you can easily see how meal planning is a great way to stick to your healthy plant-based lifestyle.

With that being said, you will be happy to find that all of the recipes can easily have ingredients swapped out or have some of your favorite foods added. The sky is the limit with the array of plant-based foods that can be put together to create delicious meals no matter where you are on your food journey or what resources you may have.

With this guide you will see that it does not have to mean cooking three meals a day, seven days a week, but if you want to do that you most certainly can! Since you are just getting started, you can still start small and work your way up, not making a meal for every day that you see on the schedule in this chapter. For example, begin with cooking dinner three to four nights a week, and work your way up from there over time. Or double (or triple) the recipe, allowing for more days to be used to have something to eat. Sometimes, this kind of planning and transitioning can be likened to a marathon, which means it is so important to pace yourself on this journey.

Something to keep close in mind when looking over this guide is that just because you set up all of your meals for the week (or month in this case), doesn't mean that you have to stick to it to the tee. It sounds like it is completely against the whole point of meal planning, doesn't it? Don't worry it really is not. Your meal plan doesn't have to be concrete. If you are not interested in chopping up a bunch of veggies to make a soup, don't fret! Throw them in a roasting pan with some plant-based oil and herbs, and 'viola!' your soup recipe is not a great addition to a Buddha Bowl! Also, scan over the Plan below and see which meals can be made to double as other meals throughout the week. For example, depending on your family size, a meal for dinner can easily be stored and eaten for lunch the next day or a different day during the week. Also, something simple for lunch can be turned into dinner by adding one additional side. The same goes with the snack and dessert recipes too! There won't be any meal shortages on this journey!

This 30-Day Meal Plan is totally flexible. There is an all-embracing structure in place to help you meet your goal of making the transition to eating plant-based a total success. As you set up your own program get ready to have that great feeling of knowing that your meals are all planned out and taken care of and you can spend more time doing the things that matter most to you. Enjoy!

Week One

Breakfast

- Cinnamon Peanut Butter Banana Overnight Oats
- Savory Sweet Potato Hash with Black Beans
- Nutty Breakfast Cookies
- Super Protein Chia Pudding
- Very Berry Smoothie
- Cinnamon Apple Muffins
- Carrot Cake-like Overnight Oats

Lunch

- Hearty Roasted Veggie Buddha Bowl
- Simple Hummus and Veggie Wrap
- Veggie Noodle Salad
- Potato and Bean Burritos
- Super Greens Avocado Salad
- Coconut Quinoa Power Bowl
- Super Easy Lentil Tacos

Dinner

- Sweet Potato and Black Bean Burger
- Warm and Hearty Stew
- Easy Beans and Rice
- Asian Tofu and Broccoli Stir Fry

- Quick Easy Burrito Bowl
- Plant-Based Creamy Chowder
- Potato and Bean Burritos

Snacks/Dessert

- Simple Sweet Potato Dip
- Easy Nice Cream

Week Two

Breakfast

- Quick Chickpea Omelet
- Fruity Muesli
- Easy Oat and Fruit Waffles
- Cinnamon Peanut Butter Banana Overnight Oats
- Savory Sweet Potato Hash with Black Beans
- Nutty Breakfast Cookies
- Super Protein Chia Pudding

Lunch

- Green Curry Cauliflower Salad
- Mediterranean Tempeh Flatbread
- Very Hearty Veggie Medley

- Spicy Nutty Tofu Lettuce Wraps
- Hearty Roasted Veggie Buddha Bowl
- Simple Hummus and Veggie Wrap
- Veggie Noodle Salad

Dinner

- Hearty Roasted Veggie Buddha Bowl
- Simple Hummus and Veggie Wrap
- Veggie Noodle Salad
- Potato and Bean Burritos
- Warm and Hearty Stew
- Quick Easy Burrito Bowl
- Plant-Based Creamy Chowder
- Spicy Nutty Tofu Lettuce Wraps

Snacks and Desserts

- Cranberry Oat Cookies
- Spicy Crispy Cauliflower

Week Three

Breakfast

- Easy Oat and Fruit Waffles
- Fruity Muesli
- Quick Chickpea Quiche

- Carrot Cake-like Overnight Oats
- Cinnamon Apple Muffins
- Very Berry Smoothie
- Super Protein Chia Pudding

Lunch

- Spicy Nutty Tofu Lettuce Wraps
- Very Hearty Veggie Medley
- Mediterranean Tempeh Flatbread
- Green Curry Cauliflower Salad
- Super Easy Lentil Tacos
- Coconut Quinoa Power Bowl
- Super Greens Avocado Salad
- Potatoes and Bean Burritos

Dinner

- Plant-Based Creamy Chowder
- Quick Easy Burrito Bowl
- Asian Tofu and Broccoli Stir Fry
- Easy Beans and Rice
- Warm and Hearty Stew
- Sweet Potato and Black Bean Burger
- Spicy Nutty Tofu Lettuce Wraps

Snacks and Dessert

- Berry Apple Crumble Bake
- Crunchy Chickpea Sticks

Week Four

Breakfast

- Very Berry Smoothie
- Quick Chickpea Quiche
- Carrot Cake-like Overnight Oats
- Cinnamon Apple Muffins
- Cinnamon Peanut Butter Banana Overnight Oats
- Savory Sweet Potato Hash with Black Beans
- Nutty Breakfast Cookies

Lunch

- Plant-Based Creamy Chowder
- Quick Easy Burrito Bowl
- Asian Tofu and Broccoli Stir Fry
- Hearty Roasted Veggie Buddha Bowl
- Simple Hummus and Veggie Wrap
- Veggie Noodle Salad
- Potato and Bean Burritos

Dinner

- Hearty Roasted Veggie Buddha Bowl

- Simple Hummus and Veggie Wrap
- Veggie Noodle Salad
- Potato and Bean Burritos
- Super Greens Avocado Salad
- Coconut Quinoa Power Bowl
- Super Easy Lentil Tacos

Snacks and Desserts

- Quick Easy Nice Cream
- Spicy Crispy Cauliflower

6

Breakfast Recipes

In this chapter, you will find all the easy-to-do and creative recipe ideas you can enjoy while taking control of your health with the Plant-Based Diet. Enjoy!

There is absolutely no shortage of great breakfast options. There are so many to choose from on a plant-based diet. Don't make breakfast too complex. You just have to really make time for doing even the most menial parts of the process. What would you do, then, in case you tend to readjust your alarm in the morning rather than get up in time to make breakfast? As you learned earlier in this book, it's possible to make all the necessary preparations in advance (i.e., prior to sleeping). In this way, you are already set for cooking breakfast. You will notice many ideas that will make this so easy to do. Because ideas for breakfast are usually the hardest to come up with, you will find a nice variety to choose from. You can make something every day as you see on the Meal Planning Guide, or you can cook a few things per week that will cover the days you need to make sure that you are eating plant-based every day.

A way to be proactive when shopping (and actually save you money) is filling up your storage with one week's worth of supplies such as:

- Whole-Grain or Sprouted Grain Breads
- Plant-Based Milk
- Whole Grain Cereals (with no added sugar or oils)
- Fruit Preserves
- Whole Grains (brown rice, millet, quinoa, etc.)
- Fresh or Frozen Fruit
- Flax Seeds
- Oats (rolled, old-fashioned, or steel-cut)

It's advisable to restock within the same week, especially in the case that a significant part of your diet entails fruits—but of course, this can be adjusted when you have frozen fruits. This practice will prove beneficial if you go big on smoothies, as ensuring the quality of the fruits to be used wouldn't be that much of a burden on your part. Bonus tip: stop at the store before your supply runs out—maybe a day or two beforehand. This way, there is no excuse!

Cinnamon Peanut Butter Banana Overnight Oats

The preparation time is 15 min. and can be served after more than 3 hours in the refrigerator.

What to Use:

- Sliced Ripe Bananas (.5 cup)
- Non-Daily Milk (one cup)
- Cinnamon (half of a teaspoon)
- Old-Fashion Oats (one cup)
- Peanut Butter (one tablespoon)

What to Do:

- Use any glass container or jar.
- Add milk, oats, and cinnamon to the container.
- Mix well. You can add more liquid or more oats depending on how thin or thick you may want it.
- Cover with lid or plastic wrap.
- Place in refrigerator for at least 3 hours.
- Add sliced bananas and peanut butter on top. Enjoy!

Savory Sweet Potato Hash with Black Beans

The preparation and cooking time is around 20 min.

What to Use:

- Black Beans (one cup cooked)
- Chopped green onions (.25 cup)

- Diced Sweet Potatoes, with or without skin (two cups)
- Chopped Onion (one cup)
- Minced Garlic (one or two cloves)
- Chili Powder (2 tsp)
- Vegetable Broth (.3 cup)
- Cilantro (for garnish)

What to Do:

- Sauté onions and garlic in non-stick skillet.
- Add one to two teaspoons of broth, and then add sweet potatoes and chili powder, Coat everything well.
- Cook until potatoes are soft and cooked through. Mix to keep from sticking by adding broth as needed.
- Add green onions and black beans. Cook until beans are heated through.
- Adjust seasoning to personal preferences.
- Serve with cilantro on top. Enjoy!

Nutty Breakfast Cookies

The preparation and cooking time is around 20 min. Can make about 12 cookies.

What to Use:

- Vanilla (one teaspoon)
- Cinnamon (one teaspoon)
- Warm filtered water (.5 cup)
- Vanilla (one teaspoon)
- Sunflower Seeds (one tablespoon)
- Maple syrup (.25 cup)
- Nut Butter (.5 cup)
- Rolled or Old Fashion Oats (two cups)
- Raisins (.25 cup)
- Chia Seeds (.2 cup)

What to Do:

- Heat oven to 350 degrees.
- Use parchment paper on a cookie sheet.
- Mix your chia seeds, warm water, and raisins. Let sit for five minutes.
- Lightly blend one cup of oats. In large bowl, add the other cup of oats with this mixture.
- Add nut butter to dry mixture. Make sure to create an even mix.
- Mix in chia/raisin and water mixture. Using a wooden spoon, blend well.
- Add sunflower seeds, maple syrup, cinnamon, and vanilla. Mix well.
- Use a scooper to scoop even amounts onto cookie sheet. Or with wet hands, form into small balls and flatten with a spoon.

- Let bake for 10 minutes. Once cool, keep in airtight container. Enjoy!

Super Protein Chia Pudding

The preparation time is around 5 min. and can be served after 2 hours. The recipe is for a single serving.

What to Use:

- Vanilla (.25 teaspoon)
- Cinnamon (.2 teaspoon)
- Cooked Quinoa (.25 cup)
- Chia Seeds (two teaspoons)
- Plant-Based Milk (.75 cup)
- Maple syrup (two teaspoons)
- Hemp Seeds for topping (optional)
- Chopped nuts for topping (optional)
- Cut up fruit for topping (optional)

What to Do:

- Mix together, chia seeds, cooked quinoa, plant-based milk, cinnamon, and maple syrup.
- Put in a glass container (small mason jar or bowl)
- Place in refrigerator and leave for about 2 hours.
- Once already set, add other nut or fruit toppings that you like. Enjoy!

Very Berry Smoothie

The preparation and serving time is around 5 min. Serves two.

What to Use:

- Plant-based Milk (two cups)
- Frozen or fresh berries (two cups of your choice)
- Frozen ripe bananas (half a cup, for sweetness)
- Flax Seeds (two teaspoons)
- Vanilla (.25 teaspoon)
- Cinnamon (.25 teaspoon)

What to Do:

- Mix together milk, flax seeds, and fruit. Blend in a high-power blender.
- Add cinnamon and vanilla. Blend until smooth.
- Serve and enjoy!

Cinnamon Apple Muffins

The preparation time is 20 min., while the cooking time is around 30 min. Makes about a dozen muffins.

What to Use:

- Apples (half a cup, peeled and chopped)
- Raisins (half a cup)

- Apple Cider Vinegar (one teaspoon)
- Plant-based Milk (.5 cup)
- Vanilla (one teaspoon)
- Cinnamon (one teaspoon)
- Apple Sauce (1.5 cups)
- Brown Sugar (.5 cup)
- All Spice (.25 teaspoon)
- Salt (.25 teaspoon)
- Baking Powder (one teaspoon)
- Baking Soda (one teaspoon)
- Whole Wheat Flour (two cups)

What to Do:

- Heat oven to 350 degrees.
- Mix together all dry ingredients into a big bowl. Set aside (flour, sugar, salt, baking powder and soda, allspice, cinnamon).
- Mix together all wet ingredients in a smaller bowl using a whisk. Set aside (apple sauce, milk, vanilla, and vinegar).
- Mix together both mixtures until smooth.
- Add apples and raisins; coat well.
- Scoop batter into silicone or non-stick muffin pan.
- Let bake for 25 minutes. Let cool. Enjoy!

Carrot Cake-Like Overnight Oats

The preparation time is around 15 min. and is ready after 3 hours in the refrigerator.

What to Use:

- Shredded carrots (.5 cup)
- Non-Daily Milk (one cup)
- Cinnamon (.25 teaspoon)
- Old-Fashion Oats (one cup)
- Pitted dates (one tablespoon)
- Nutmeg (.25 teaspoon)
- Grated or dried Ginger (.3 teaspoon)
- Vanilla (.25 teaspoon)
- Hemp Seeds (.25 teaspoon)

What to Do:

- Use any glass container or jar.
- Add all ingredients together in a container.
- Mix well. You can add more liquid or more oats depending on how thin or thick you may want it.
- Cover with lid or plastic wrap.
- Place in refrigerator for at least 3 hours.
- Once set, mix together. Enjoy!

Fruity Muesli

The preparation and serving time is around 5 min.

What to Use:

- Plant-Based Milk (.5 cup)
- Maple Syrup (two teaspoons)
- Chopped Nuts (.25 cup)
- Dried Fruit (.5 cup)
- Freeze Dried Fruit (one cup)
- Rolled Oats (1 cup)

What to Do:

- In a bowl mix together milk, maple syrup, oats, fruit, and nuts.
- Add milk to eat immediately like cereal.
- Add milk and refrigerate for an overnight version.
- Enjoy!

Easy Oat and Waffles

The preparation and serving time is around 30 min. Makes about 10 waffles.

What to Use:

- Ripe Mashed Bananas (.3 cup)
- Cinnamon (.5 teaspoon)
- Flax Seeds (.25 cup ground)
- Unsweetened Almond Milk (.5 cup)
- Rolled Oats (2 cups)
- Lemon Zest (2 teaspoons)
- Sliced Bananas and Strawberries (2 cups)

What to Do:

- Using a food processor, mix oats, flax seeds, cinnamon, and lemon zest. Form a powder.
- Add milk and mashed bananas to make a thick batter.
- Using a preheated waffle iron add some of the batter and close lid.
- Repeat until finish batter. Top with fresh sliced fruit. Enjoy!

Quick Chickpea Omelet

The preparation and cooking time is around 30 min. Makes about 3–5 omelets.

What to Use:

- Chopped mushrooms (.25 cup sautéed)
- Green Onions (.5 cup)
- Baking Soda (.5 teaspoon)
- Nutritional Yeast (.3 cup)
- Black Pepper (.25 teaspoon)
- White Pepper (.25 teaspoon)
- Garlic Powder (.5 teaspoon)
- Onion Powder (.5 teaspoon)
- Chickpea Flour (one cup)

What to Do:

- In a small bowl mix together: Baking soda, yeast, both types of pepper, garlic powder, onion powder, and chickpea flour.
- Add one cup of water to the mixture and mix well. Make a smooth batter.
- Heat up a non-stick skillet. Add plant-based oil if desired.
- Using the same method as making pancakes, do add batter into the pan.
- Add green onions and mushrooms in the middle of the omelet.
- Flip twice once each side is a golden brown color.
- Let it cool. Enjoy!

7

Lunch Recipes

I n this chapter, you will find all the easy-to-do and creative recipe ideas you can enjoy while taking control of your health with the Plant-Based Diet. Enjoy!

When it comes to planning lunch, it is usually better to go with what is more convenient and something that can easily be stored in to-go containers. As always, the focus is to make sure you have whatever meal you need for those moments when you are ready to eat! This way, you will not be tempted when the usual Pizza Shop menu gets passed around the office or when that smell of French fries catches you as you drive past a fast food place.

We have all been there! However, it doesn't have to end with resetting your journey to eat plant-based every day!

There are a few ways to make this a success:

Double or Triple Up: You may have noticed what types of easy recipes are in this book for lunch. As you look over the ingredients and the quantities, you can easily adjust to make more. You may find that you to cook up a bigger portion and then portion out single servings in nice airtight containers once or twice a week. This way, you can keep them in the refrigerator and take out for whichever day you need. A really great additional option is to cook up your favorite high protein grain and portion that out to add to your lunch meal.

Take the leftovers from last night's meal: One great thing that you will see in both the lunch and dinner meals is that they are interchangeable. So don't worry too much about what you will eat the next day, especially if you had such a great dinner the night before. The beauty of plant-based meals is that their fresh ingredients can really be eaten any time of day, without that gross "overly full" feeling. So no falling asleep at your desk after lunch!

Another great thing that can be done in advance is to look over your menu and select something you can double up as your lunch for the next day. Then while prepping the family dinner, you can kill two birds with one "pot" and set aside tomorrow's lunch. This may even help give you a little more time to watch another episode of your favorite show before bed, rather than making lunches.

Salads are always easy: At the end of the day, your goal with this diet is to eat more plant-based foods. This can easily be done by prepping plant foods to go with you, and actually become the meal of that time. Such as just cutting up some cucumbers, carrots, Brussels or radishes and place them into a go container. Mix up a bunch of your favorite greens and have them stored in the fridge as well for easy access. You can have some beans, or grains, or roasted veggies in airtight containers that are easy to grab and throw on those greens. Whichever methods you chose you won't have to worry about not having the means to eat well! Bonus tip: Ensuring that your ingredients are separated from another will aid in maintaining their freshness.

Hearty Roasted Veggie Buddha Bowl

The preparation time is 10 min., while the cooking time is around 20 min.

What to Use:

- Cooked Brown Rice (one cup)
- Brussel Sprouts (four cups)
- Sliced Carrots (two cups)
- Plant-Based Oil (two teaspoons)
- Broccoli cuts (one cup)
- Salt and Pepper
- Minced Garlic (one clove)
- Lemon Juice (half a lemon)
- Tahini (.25 cup)
- Water (.25)

What to Do:

- Heat oven to 450 degrees.
- Blend together tahini, lemon juice, water, and garlic. Set sauce aside.
- In another bowl, coat chopped vegetables with plant-based oil.
- Lay across the cookie sheet. Sprinkle salt and pepper evenly on all vegetables.
- Let cook in the oven for about twenty minutes.
- Layer cooked rice and roasted vegetables. Drizzle on the sauce to taste. Enjoy!

Simple Hummus and Veggie Wrap

The preparation and serving time is around 20 min.

What to Use:

- Homemade or pre-made hummus (four tablespoons)
- Non-dairy plain yogurt (two teaspoons)
- Broccoli Slaw (.5 cup)
- Fresh Lime Juice (two teaspoons)
- Thinly Sliced Apples (.25 cups)
- Salt and Pepper
- Whole Grain Tortillas
- Leafy lettuce of your choice.

What to Do:

- Place in a bowl the broccoli slaw, lime juice, and yogurt. Mix well.
- Evenly spread hummus on tortilla.
- Layer lettuce, apple slices, and slaw on the tortilla.
- Fold the tortilla up like a burrito. (Fold up the bottom, tuck in one side, and roll.)
- Cut in two pieces. Use extra hummus to dip. Enjoy!

Veggie Noodle Salad

The preparation and serving time is around 20 min.

What to Use:

- Jarred Artichokes (.25 cup chopped)
- Red Onion (one teaspoon chopped)
- Cherry Tomatoes (.5 cup chopped)
- Half of a Yellow Pepper Sliced Thin
- Half of a Red Pepper Sliced Thin
- Spiralizer Cucumber (two English)
- Spiralizer Zucchini (two)
- Mint Leaves (chopped)
- Olive Oil (.5 tablespoon)
- Red Wine Vinegar (1.5 tablespoons)
- Salt (.25 teaspoon)
- Italian Seasoning (one teaspoon)
- Garlic Powder (.25 teaspoon)

What to Do:

- Put spiralizer cucumber and zucchini in a bowl.
- In another bowl, add seasoning, red wine vinegar, olive oil, and chopped mint. Mix well.
- Add to sliced peppers, coat evenly.
- Layer your spiralizer veggies and peppers in a bowl or container with the lid.
- Add your favorite plant-based protein. Enjoy!

Potatoes and Bean Burritos

The preparation and serving time is around 20 min.

What to Use:

- Cooked Beans of your choice (.25 cup chopped)
- Vegetable Broth (.5 cup)
- Olive Oil (.5 tablespoon)
- Garlic Cloves (three to five minced)
- Salt and Pepper
- Onion (.5 cup diced)
- Ten of your Favorite Kind of Potato (peeled and chopped small)
- Warm tortillas

What to Do:

- Cook potatoes in oil and veggie broth with garlic and onions in a skillet.
- Once potatoes are soft, add beans and stir to keep from sticking to the pan. Add more liquid if needed.
- Layer cooked mixture on tortilla.
- Top it with plant-based salsa and hot sauce.
- Fold burrito style. Enjoy!

Super Greens Avocado Salad

The preparation and serving time is around 20 min.

What to Use:

- Mixed Greens (one handful)
- Chopped Avocado (two small)
- Chickpeas (cooked one cup)
- Olive Oil (two tbsp.)
- Apple Cider Vinegar (1 tbsp.)
- Cilantro (2 tbsp.)
- Lime juice
- Minced shallots (one tablespoon)
- Dijon Mustard (one tablespoon)
- Chopped Cucumber (one cup)

What to Do:

- Put shallots, mustard, cilantro, lime juice and zest, and vinegar together in a bowl. Slowly whisk in oil.
- Combine with chickpeas and cucumbers. Coat well.
- Line a bowl with greens.
- Add veggie mixture.
- Top with avocado. Drizzle more dressing. Enjoy!

Coconut Quinoa Power Bowl

The preparation time is 10 min., while the cooking time is around 20 min.

What to Use:

- Cooked Quinoa (one cup)
- Cooked Black Beans (one cup)
- Sweet Potatoes (two cups peeled and chopped)
- Plant-Based Oil (two teaspoons)
- Chopped Red Peppers (one cup)
- Salt and Pepper
- Minced Garlic (one clove)
- Lemon Juice (half a lemon)
- Onions (.25 cup)
- Coconut Milk (.25 cup)
- Lime Juice (one teaspoon)
- Olive Oil (one teaspoon)
- Agave (one tablespoon)

What to Do:

- Heat oven to 450 degrees.
- Mix together agave, olive oil. Lime juice, and coconut milk. Set aside.
- Roast sweet potatoes, garlic, and peppers, on cookie sheet.
- Layer your quinoa, black beans, and roasted veggies in a bowl.
- Pour dressing over the contents. Add in your condiments according to your preference. Enjoy!

Super-Easy Lentil Tacos

The preparation time is 10 min., while the cooking time is around 20 min.

What to Use:

- Corn Tortillas
- Mashed Avocado (one cup)
- Chopped Cilantro (one tablespoon)
- Plant-Based Oil (two teaspoons)
- Diced Tomatoes (.25 cup)
- Taco Seasoning (Cumin, Garlic Powder, Chili Powder, Salt, and Pepper)
- Lettuce (a handful of your choice)
- Lime Juice (half a lime squeezed; slice another half)
- Dry Lentils (one cup)

- Hot Sauce (optional)

What to Do:

- In a small saucepan, put lentils with two cups of water, oil, and lime juice. Cook until soft. About 15 minutes.
- Drain rest of water in beans. Season it with taco seasoning.
- Layer your beans with mashed avocados, tomatoes, lettuce and cilantro in warmed corn tortillas.
- Add hot sauce and extra lime juice if desired. Enjoy!

Green Curry Cauliflower Salad

The preparation and serving time is around 25 min.

What to Use:

- Mixed Greens of your choice (five cups)
- Cauliflower (three cups)
- Chopped Cilantro (one tablespoon)
- Red Grapes (one cup halved)
- Cooked lentils (one cup)
- Melted Coconut Oil (1.5 tablespoons)
- Tahini (two tablespoons)
- Lemon Juice (two tablespoons)
- Curry Paste (4.5 tablespoons)

- Curry Powder (1.5 tablespoons)
- Maple Syrup (one tablespoon)
- Salt (.25 teaspoon)

What to Do:

- Heat oven to 400 degrees. Prepare a baking sheet with parchment paper.
- Put chopped cauliflower in a bowl, add coconut oil, curry powder, and salt. Put on baking sheet and bake until golden color.
- In a small bowl put paste, tahini, lemon juice, maple syrup, and salt; blend well using a whisk.
- Layer your greens with cooked lentils, cauliflower, and grapes in a container with a lid.
- Add curry dressing to the salad. Cover and shake to evenly distribute dressing.
- Top with cilantro. Enjoy!

Mediterranean Tempeh Flatbread

The preparation and serving time is around 35 min.

What to Use:

- Silken Tofu (.75 cup)
- Whole Grain Flatbread Wraps
- Red Onion Sliced (.5 cup)
- Tomatoes Sliced (.5 cup)

- White Wine Vinegar (.5 teaspoon)
- Chopped Dill (1 tablespoon)
- Cucumber (.5 cup peeled and shredded)
- Lemon Juice (one tablespoon)
- Coconut Amino Acids or Reduced Sodium Soy Sauce (two tablespoons)
- Yellow Onion (.25 cup)
- Olive Oil (one tablespoon)
- Thinly Sliced Tempeh (one-eight-ounce package)

What to Do:

- Heat skillet with oil on medium heat. Lay sliced tempeh in oil. Brown on both sides.
- Mix in a bowl the onions, garlic, and soy sauce/coconut amino. Season with favorite Italian herbs. Add a half of cup of water to help coat.
- Add this mixture to tempeh. Lower heat and let cook about 10 minutes.
- Put tofu and garlic in high-speed blender. Mix in cucumber, lemon juice, dill, and vinegar.
- Layer your tempeh, spread, onions, and tomatoes on flatbread.
- Sprinkle with salt and pepper if needed. Enjoy!

Very Hearty Veggie Medley

The preparation and serving time is around 45 min. This serves about four to five people.

What to Use:

- Garlic Cloves (two minced)
- Sliced Sweet Potatoes (two cups)
- Parsley (.25 teaspoon)
- Purple Sweet Potato (one cup)
- Vegetable Broth (.25 cup)
- Summer Squash Sliced (one cup)
- Sliced Carrots (one cup)
- Plant Oil (two tablespoons)
- Salt and Pepper (one teaspoon each)
- Chopped Onion (one cup)
- Brussel Sprouts (one cup halved)
- Oregano (one tablespoon)
- Sage (one teaspoon)
- Rosemary (one teaspoon)
- Chili Powder (one tablespoon)
- Maple Syrup (one tablespoon)

What to Do:

- Heat oven to 400 degrees.
- Coat chopped vegetables with oil, salt, and pepper. Put in a single layer on cookie sheet. Bake for 35 minutes.
- In a small bowl, mix maple syrup, oil, chili powder, rosemary, sage, oregano, and broth together.

- Toss roasted vegetables with broth mix. Put back in the oven for 10 minutes.
- Serve by itself or with your favorite protein side. Enjoy!

Spicy Nutty Tofu Lettuce Wraps

The preparation and serving time is around 35 min.

What to Use:

- Extra Firm Tofu (one container)
- Nut Butter (.5 cup)
- Brown rice noodles (two cups)
- Ginger (one teaspoon)
- Rice Vinegar (.25 cup)
- Sesame Oil (.3 cup)
- Garlic (one clove minced)
- Chili Paste (two tablespoons)
- Cilantro (one teaspoon)
- Agave (two teaspoons)
- Low Sodium Soy Sauce (.3 cups)
- Large Lettuce Leaves

What to Do:

- Prepare noodles in lukewarm water to make soft and flexible.
- Put together agave, chili paste, ginger, soy sauce,

rice vinegar, sesame oil, garlic, and nut butter in a blender. Mix well.

- Warm oil in a skillet and sauté tofu. Add half of the sauce mix. Put in the bowl on the side.
- Add more oil to hot pan and add drained noodles. Add to tofu.
- Add mixture to lettuce leaves and top with cilantro. Roll up. Enjoy!

8

Dinner Recipes

In this chapter, you will find all the easy-to-do and creative recipe ideas you can enjoy while taking control of your health with the Plant-Based Diet. Enjoy!

Many times throughout this book, you have read that each person is different in how they go about making this transition a success. A simple way to add to that is having the comfort of knowing the answer to the question: "What's for dinner?" You can easily adjust to doing what works for you and your family. One way to do that may be to prepare your meals on the weekend. Some have found success in cooking all the meals for the week and having them stored for easy access. When doing this, keep in mind that it will lessen your stress if you make sure to shop accordingly. This may mean doing a quick inventory before heading to the store so that you don't find yourself buying what you don't even need, or even worse, not getting that key ingredient. Another great thing to do when planning in advance is thinking ahead as to what kind of schedule you have for that particular week. Are you in back-to-back meetings at work meant to drain your mental faculties and make you opt for a run through the drive through? Do the kids have playoff games 4 times during the week? Do you have family coming for a visit? These and so many other scenarios can adversely affect what you may want to cook versus what you should cook to stay on track. Hence, get ahead of them!

Another way is to notice the ingredients a meal calls for. As you may have noticed, many of the sample recipes have some of the same easy ingredients. Can you plan accordingly to make meals with these foods every week? Because you will most definitely be tapping into your creative side, don't worry about whether or not you will be eating the same things. With the abundance of flavors that come with a plant-based diet, you will soon see that one ingredient in one recipe tastes completely different in another. Also, you will see that the recipes can easily swap out different ingredients. Are you tired of black beans? Switch it up for pinto beans? Need a little more color? Use orange and yellow bell peppers instead of green and red. So many choices are right at your fingertips to have you diving in for seconds!

And finally, with all of this advanced cooking or day of cooking, make sure to keep your cooking space comfortable. Don't shop at a wholesale store if you don't have the extra storage. This will only cause stress and not encourage a fun cooking environment. Keep in mind, what is on sale too and swap out those ingredients. This, of course, will save lots of money, but it will also help you to see how you can immediately get creative in your recipes, which in turn create even more meals. Along with the specific food ingredients, you will see that there are other condiments that are common throughout the recipe. This is such a great bonus because how many of us have bought a 15-ounce jar of pickled artichoke hearts for a recipe that only necessitated a quarter of a cup—only to have them thrown out in your refrigerator cleanup day? Yeah, we don't want that to happen. Hence, keep that in mind with your future recipes. Be aware of what you have, and change it up, whenever you can!

Sweet Potato and Black Bean Burger

The preparation and serving time is around 40 min. Serves about 4–5.

What to Use:

- Shiitake Mushrooms (2 cups)
- Plant-Based Mayonnaise (.25 cup)
- Soy Sauce (1.5 tablespoons)
- Shelled Sunflower Seeds (.5 cup)
- Cooked Black Beans (1.5 cups)
- Green Onions (two stalks)
- Old Fashion Oats (.75 cup)
- Boiled Sweet Potato (two cups mashed)

- Salt and Pepper (.5 teaspoon)
- Garlic Powder (.5 teaspoon)
- Smoked Paprika (.5 teaspoon)
- Mirin (1.5 tablespoons)
- Sriracha (one teaspoon)

What to Do:

- Place oats, mashed sweet potato, beans, sunflower seeds, onions, salt and pepper, garlic powder, paprika, soy sauce and mirin in a bowl. Using hands mix well. Make sure beans are mashed and blended.
- Heat oven to 375 degrees. Put parchment paper on a baking sheet.
- Form your mixture into patties, then put them on the sheet. Then, bake for 20 minutes on each side.
- While patties are cooking, slice mushrooms and sauté in olive oil, soy sauce, and mirin. Then, cook for about one minute.
- Make a sauce out of mayo and Sriracha. Make with more hot sauce to taste.
- Serve on your favorite whole grain or gluten-free bun. Top with mushrooms, sauce mixture, and your favorite greens. Enjoy!

Warm and Hearty Stew

The preparation and serving time is around 60 min. Serves has about four to five servings.

What to Use:

- Spinach (three cups)
- Garbanzo Beans (one can – drained)
- Vegetable Broth (two cups)
- Diced Tomatoes (one can – drained)
- Sliced Sweet Potatoes (five cups)
- Minced Garlic (three cloves)
- Chopped Onions (one cup)
- Cooked Quinoa (two cups)
- Olive Oil (two tablespoons)
- Paprika (one teaspoon)
- Cumin (one teaspoon)
- Coriander (.5 teaspoon)
- Turmeric (.5 teaspoon)
- Ground Ginger (.5 teaspoon)
- Cinnamon (.5 teaspoon)
- Cayenne Pepper (pinch)
- Chopped Cilantro (two tablespoons)
- Lemon slices (for garnish)
- Non-dairy Yogurt (optional garnish)

What to Do:

- Heat a large pot with olive oil. Sauté garlic, onions for about five minutes.

- Add all seasonings and mix well.
- Put broth in the pot, then add in your tomatoes. Mix well. Bring to boil.
- Add sweet potatoes and beans.
- Lower heat to make simmer for about 30 minutes.
- Turn heat off, add spinach. Let cook for another two minutes.
- Serve in a small bowl topped with cilantro, squeezed lemon juice, and a teaspoon of non-dairy yogurt. Enjoy!

Easy Beans and Rice

The preparation and serving time is around 35 min.

What to Use:

- Plant-Based Broth (one cup)
- Red Kidney Beans (two cans drained)
- Diced Tomatoes (one can)
- Plant-based Oil (two tablespoons)
- Chopped Garlic (four cloves)
- Chopped Green Pepper (.5 cup)
- Chopped Celery (.5 cup)
- Chopped Yellow Onions (one cup)
- Cooked Brown Rice (four cups)
- Cayenne Pepper (.5 teaspoon)
- Dried Italian Herbs (two teaspoons)
- Two Bay Leaves

- Salt and Pepper
- Chopped Parsley (garnish topping)
- Hot Sauce (optional)

What to Do:

- In a large pot, put your olive oil, onions, celery, peppers, and garlic. Sauté for about one to two minutes.
- Add the broth, beans, and tomatoes. Sprinkle in cayenne pepper, paprika, Italian herbs, bay leaves, salt, and pepper.
- Let cook on low for about 15 to 20 minutes. Let sauce thicken.
- Once cooked, remove bay leaves.
- Warm cooked brown rice.
- Serve both in a small bowl topped with parsley and hot sauce. Enjoy!

Asian Tofu and Broccoli Stir Fry

The preparation and serving time is around 45 min. Serves about four.

What to Use:

- Plant-Based Broth (.25 cup)
- Minced Ginger (three tablespoons)
- Cornstarch (two teaspoons)

- Red Pepper Flakes (one teaspoon)
- Chopped Garlic (two cloves)
- Coconut Oil (one tablespoon)
- Broccoli Cuts (four cups)
- Extra firm Tofu (one package cut into cubes)
- Cooked grain of your choice (brown rice, quinoa, barley, etc.)
- Coconut Amino Acids/Low Sodium Soy Sauce (.3 cup)
- Rice Wine Vinegar (one tablespoon)
- Sesame Oil (two tablespoons)

What to Do:

- In a small bowl add amino acids or soy sauce, vinegar, sesame oil, garlic, ginger, red pepper flakes, broth, and corn starch. Use a whisk to mix well. Sit to the side.
- Set oven to 400 degrees.
- In a different bowl, coat your broccoli and tofu with sauce mixture. Put in a single layer on a baking sheet.
- Put the contents into the oven and cook for about 20 minutes or until tofu is golden and crisp.
- Warm cooked brown rice.
- In small pot, heat your sauce until it gets thick. Let cool

- Serve tofu and broccoli on top of rice. Add sauce to taste. Enjoy!

Quick Easy Burrito Bowl

The preparation and serving time is around 20 min. Serves about four to five.

What to Use:

- Chili Powder (.5 teaspoon)
- Cumin (one teaspoon)
- Lime Juice (one tablespoon)
- Vegan Sour Cream (.25 cup)
- Smashed Avocado (one small)
- Chopped Cilantro (a handful)
- Diced Red Bell Pepper (one cup)
- Salsa (your choice of one jar)
- Cooked Brown Rice or Favorite Grain (two cups)
- Corn (two cups canned or frozen)
- Cooked Black Beans (one can – drained)

What to Do:

- Cook rice or grains as directed.
- In a small bowl put smashed avocado, cumin, chili powder, vegan sour cream, and lime juice. Blend well. Put to the side.
- Once rice is cooked put in black beans, salsa, and

corn. Cook together for about five minutes, stir to mix well.

- Turning off heat, add peppers and cilantro and mix well.
- Serve the rice and vegetable mix in a bowl. Add dressing to taste. Enjoy!

Plant-Based Creamy Chowder

The preparation and serving time is around 40 min. Serves about four to five.

What to Use:

- Garlic Cloves (two minced)
- Corn Kernels (two cups)
- Fresh Dill (.25 teaspoon)
- Purple Sweet Potato (one chopped in small pieces)
- Vegetable Broth (.25 cup)
- Coconut Milk (one can)
- Plant Oil (two tablespoons)
- Salt and Pepper (one teaspoon each)
- Chopped Onion (one cup)
- Cooked Quinoa (one cup)
- Oregano (one tablespoon)
- Sage (one teaspoon)
- Rosemary (one teaspoon)
- Ginger (one tablespoon)
- Marjoram (one tablespoon)

- Thyme (one tablespoon)

What to Do:

- Cook quinoa as directed. Set aside.
- Heat oven to 400 degrees.
- Coat chopped potatoes with oil, salt, and pepper. Put in a single layer on cookie sheet. Bake for 15 minutes. Set aside.
- In a non-stick skillet put oil, onions, garlic, and celery on medium heat. Sauté for two minutes.
- Add broth, coconut milk, all spices, and corn to a saucepan on medium heat. Add mix from skillet. Let cook for ten minutes.
- Serve in soup bowls. Add a small scoop of potatoes and quinoa in chowder. Enjoy!

9

Snack Recipes

In this chapter, you will find all the easy-to-do and creative recipe ideas you can enjoy while taking control of your health with the Plant-Based Diet. Enjoy!

Do not underestimate the importance of planning your snacks, especially if you are inclined to get hungry and snack amidst your main dishes. This is pretty normal, though—you can learn how to make sure you have healthy options. It may be best to just anticipate for this to happen, to be on the safe side. This way, you will routinely keep yourself stocked with fruit, vegetables, or some kind of dip and crackers. Make sure to carry something—anything plant-based, of course—with you so that you are less likely to be faced with eating unhealthy snacks when you are out and about.

The beauty with any snacks is you can choose them based on your energy needs and the time between your next meal. Some of us have the habit of snacking out of boredom rather than hunger. If this is the case, try to have raw produce in lieu of calorie-concentrated choices that are relatively more difficult to manage.

Besides the recipes, here are some quick and easy options:

- Fresh sliced fruit:
- Berries
- Apples
- Bananas
- Melon
- Oranges
- Raw veggies:
- Carrots
- Celery
- Peppers
- Broccoli
- Cauliflower
- Summer Squash
- Zucchini
- Cold potato or sweet potato chunks or slices
- Grilled corn on the cob (it's actually really good cold!)
- Pumpkin seeds
- Sunflower seeds
- Raw almonds

- Walnuts
- Raw cashews
- Brown rice cakes
- Whole-grain or sprouted grain toast
- Dried figs
- Dates
- Homemade dips:
- Salsa
- Bean Dip
- Hummus

Simple Sweet Potato Dip

The preparation and serving time is around 10 min.

What to Use:

- Ground Cumin (one teaspoon)
- Salt and Pepper (one teaspoon)
- Lemon Juice (.75 cup)
- Garlic (2 cloves)
- Tahini (.25 cup)
- Sweet Potato Mash (one cup)

What to Do:

- Put sweet potatoes, garlic, tahini, cumin and salt,

and pepper in a food processor.
- Puree mixture completely. Season to taste.
- Serve with your favorite veggies, plant-based chips, or toast. Enjoy!

Crunchy Chickpea Sticks

The preparation and serving time is around 55 min.

What to Use:

- Butternut Squash (one cup cooked and smashed)
- Chickpeas (one can – drained)
- Cooked Brown Rice (one cup)
- Finely Chopped Onions (.25 cup)
- Nutritional Yeast (two tablespoons)
- Panko or fine bread crumbs (.5 cup)
- Salt and Pepper (one teaspoon)
- Fresh Sage (1.5 teaspoons)
- Garlic (one minced clove)
- Chopped Parsley (one tablespoon)
- Lime Juice (one tablespoon)

What to Do:

- Set oven to 350 degrees. Put parchment paper in a cookie sheet.
- Put your squash, chickpeas, and cooked rice in a

food processor. Add garlic, sage, lime juice, parsley, yeast, and onion. Blend well.

- Line bottom a small dish with panko or bread crumbs.
- Scoop about a tablespoon of mixture and make into rectangular shapes. Roll in crumb mix.
- Line forms on cookie sheet. Repeat until finish mix.
- Put in oven for about 35 minutes.
- Serve with your favorite dipping sauce or plant-based ketchup. Enjoy!

Spicy Crispy Cauliflower

The preparation and serving time is around 55 min.

What to Use:

- One head of Cauliflower (Florets separated from stems)
- Smoked Paprika (two teaspoons)
- Onion Powder (two teaspoons)
- Garlic Powder (two teaspoons)
- Tomato Paste (one tablespoon)
- Spicy Barbeque or Buffalo Sauce (.25 cup)
- Almond Flour (two tablespoons)
- Rice Flour (.5 cup)

What to Do:

- Set oven to 450 degrees. Put parchment paper in a cookie sheet.
- Put all flours, tomato paste, parsley, garlic and onion, powder, and other seasonings in a food processor with .25 cup of water. Bring the contents into a smooth batter. Add more water as needed.
- In a large bowl, mix together batter mix, and cauliflower florets. Ensuring are evenly coated.
- Fill the cookie sheet with the mixture. Spreading out evenly.
- Put in oven for about 25 minutes. Edges should be crispy. Let sit for about five minutes.
- Put in a large bowl and mix with favorite spicy barbeque sauce or buffalo sauce. Enjoy!

10

Dessert Recipes

Having a Desserts section makes so much sense when you are trying to make this a lifestyle change. For many, learning how to make desserts without using refined sugar is paramount and life-changing. Doing your research, you may have found that there are so many health problems that center on the consumption of *just* refined sugar. Hence, to boot, the plant-based diet helps get rid of that risk. Yet, does that really mean that we have to give up the joy of fulfilling our sweet tooth? No way! The key is whether baking with or just consuming something sweet, make sure that it is plant-based. You can easily research some of the alternatives, depending on your taste. Yet, in this journey, also try to discover what whole foods make for great sweets. In the recipes in this book, you will easily see how you can still enjoy your favorite treats without sacrificing your health! As with the other recipes, these can be a base for some decadent dessert creations!

Berry Apple Crumble Bake

The preparation time is around 15 min., while the baking time is around 35 min.

What to Use:

- Old Fashion Oats (two cups)
- Oat Flour (two cups)
- Frozen Berries (five cups thawed)
- Sweet Apples Peeled and Chopped (eight cups)
- Sea Salt (.25 teaspoon)
- Almond Butter (.25 cup)
- Pure Maple Syrup (.5 cup)
- Baking Powder (two teaspoons)

What to Do:

- Set oven to 425 degrees.
- Warm up chopped apples in a medium pot with a little water to keep from sticking. Cook until soft.
- Put cooked apples in a rectangular or square baking pan.
- Layer your berries on top of apple mix. Spreading evenly.
- Mix together oats, flour, maple syrup, salt, baking

powder and almond butter in a bowl. Swish together with fingers.

- Put crumble mixture on all of the fruit in pan. Then, bake for about 15–20 minutes.
- Let cool. Serve with a favorite non-daily whipped cream topping or Nice Cream. Enjoy!

Cranberry Oat Cookies

The preparation time is around 20 min., while the baking time is around 45 min.

What to Use:

- Rolled Oats (.5 cup)
- Dried Cranberries (1.5 cups)
- Tahini (.25 cup)
- Maple Syrup (.3 cup)
- Pumpkin (one can)
- Allspice (one teaspoon)
- Nutmeg (one teaspoon)
- Cinnamon (two teaspoons)
- Baking Powder (four teaspoons)
- Cornmeal (one cup)

What to Do:

- Heat oven to 350 degrees.

- Put cornmeal, baking powder, salt, nutmeg, cinnamon, and allspice in a small bowl.
- In a larger bowl, put tahini, maple syrup, and pumpkin. Blend together. Add other mix and blend together. Add cranberries and oats.
- Take out a small spoonful of mixture and place on a baking sheet. Using a small spoon, press down the contents to make small circles.
- Place in oven and bake for 45 minutes. Let cool for an additional ten minutes.
- Enjoy with your favorite plant-based milk. Enjoy!

Quick Easy Nice Cream

The preparation and serving time is around 50 min.

What to Use:

- Almond Milk (.5 cup)
- Frozen Bananas (about 3 cups)
- Coconut Oil (.25 cup)
- Salt (pinch)
- Cocoa or Vanilla Powder (.25 cup)

What to Do:

- In a small bowl, use a whisk to blend cocoa or vanilla powder. Make sure it is nice and smooth.

- Put bananas, almond milk, and flavor mixture into a food processor or blender.
- Using a spatula take out mixture and put into a small loaf baking pan.
- Freeze covered until ready to serve.
- Serve with all your favorite toppings. Enjoy!

Conclusion

Thank you for making it through to the end of *Plant-Based Diet: Delicious Recipes to Lose Weight, Reduce Inflammation, Reverse Disease, and Feel Great*!

The hope is that it was informative and able to provide you with all of the tools you need to achieve your goals of making a plant-based diet a part of your lifestyle.

As you carefully considered each chapter of this book, we hope that you were able to see the benefits of a Plant-Based Diet. You were able to get the confidence boost you needed to be successful in this transition. You learned exactly what you would be eating and also what you will want to avoid. This hopefully made those trips to the grocery store and market enjoyable. You learned what each category of whole foods you want to keep handy while learning how different whole foods can give you the nutrients you need on a daily basis. You have experienced what it is like to load up your shopping cart with varied delicious fresh foods to make creative and simple meals for the whole family. You learned the importance of avoiding the many common food mistakes that make people quit. You found that this journey is one that can be adjusted to you and your circumstances. That's all there is to know about sticking to it—even when it gets tough. You learned how to create the support and motivation that's needed to keep going. You took on the challenge of adapting your everyday schedule to this wonderful new lifestyle—not letting yourself be worried about what to cook next.

No one can make us make changes in our habits, especially when it comes to eating. Yet, when it is important to get a grip on our physical health, sometimes, a second opinion is warranted. We hope that this book gave you such an opinion.

You learned that a meal plan doesn't have to be scary but an enjoyable adventure that allows you to tap into your creative side in the kitchen. You were able to create an environment that encouraged healthy eating no matter what meal of the day it was—even dessert! You held on to get a good grip not only on setting yourself up for new healthy food choices but also on feeling great as well!

With all of the options and diet choices circling us every day, we hope that you have seen the benefits of choosing a Plant-Based Diet as your gateway to a healthier *you*!

The next step is to keep going! You learned key steps to making this a lifestyle change—not just a fad. You learned that you aren't perfect—so as long as you put forth every effort, every day, you can take control of your well-being. It will take time to stay balanced with a new eating habit, but the rewards will be worth it!

Finally, if you found this book useful in any way, a review on Amazon is always appreciated!

Lightning Source UK Ltd.
Milton Keynes UK
UKHW020641020622
403888UK00010B/1049

9 781087 863832